LEAN OPERATING ROOMS

Improving Operating Room Efficiency a Team Approach

RICHARD B. SILVER, MD, MBA

CreateSpace eStore: https://www.createspace.com/3712655

Amazon.com

Lean Operating Rooms

Authored by Richard B. Silver MD MBA

A Multidisciplinary Team Approach Using Lean Techniques To Improve Operating Room Efficiency

ISBN/EAN13:

1467907413 / 9781467907415

Lean Operating Rooms

DEDICATED TO MY CHILDREN

TRENT AARON SILVER

&

CLAUDIA ROSE SILVER

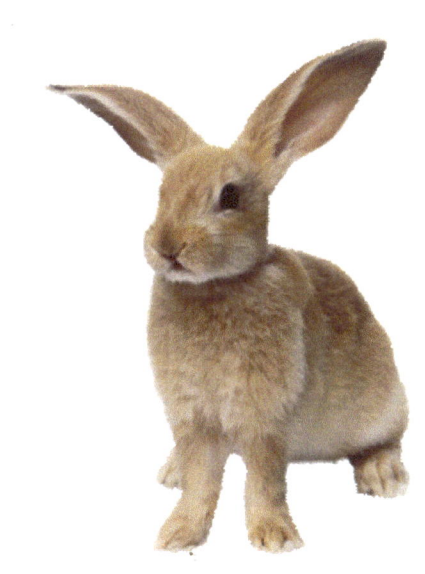

Table of Contents

ACKNOWLEDGEMENTS

I wish to thank Dr. Peter Bath for his kind assistance and support throughout this Lean project. A common quote from team members this year before our meetings was, "Will Peter be there?" He was the glue for the team and a mentor to me.

I was particularly grateful to John Dietrick, MD and his "Lean Team 6" composed of Chris Weber, RN, Rick Gonzalez, First Assist, and Yudit Conrado, Scrub Tech for their enthusiasm, honesty and willingness to make a contribution to our project. I would like to thank Jackie VanCleave, Anesthesia Assistant, and Mary Horsman, Certified Registered Nurse Anesthetist for their contribution to the team, as well as Charles Beckenstein, MD, Anesthesiologist and Lashea Lockhart, Anesthesia Administrative Assistant for coordinating the anesthesia coverage for the Lean study.

I appreciate Jan Bradley, RN, Team Leader CVOR, for her kind assistance with another Lean project in the heart surgery program, and Heather Outen, RN, and Vickie Lewis, RN for helping me with a separate Lean Registration project.

Since I "grew up" in the sciences, I have always been a little dubious of my writing skills. I want to thank my dynamic duo, "Lindas", communication educators at the Physicians Executive MBA Program at The University of Tennessee (PEMBA). Both Dr. Linda Lyle and Linda Walsh extended their patience with me this past year "tolerating" my writing skills as I tried to understand their "track changes." ☺

The PEMBA faculty has been incredible. Dr. Chuck Noon and Jody Crane, MD MBA taught me most of what I know about Lean Healthcare and then some. I was especially appreciative of Dr. Noon being patient with me when I completed my Lean Organization Action Project in a Power Point format, and kindly asking me to re-submit in a word document with a two week grace period-whew! The on campus Lean simulations they demonstrated opened my eyes to the complexities of a Lean process improvement.

Don Lighter, MD MBA was very supportive and gave me loads of time with Six Sigma and Lean analysis of my data. I appreciate his patience with my never ending barrage of questions on control charts and data analysis. There were two gratifying moments in my interaction with Don: 1) I caught a mistake in one of his p charts ☺ and 2) He referred to me as "grasshopper" in one of my aha moments-doesn't take much to make me happy. ☺

I wish to thank Dr. Ray Husband from the PEMBA faculty for helping me with my goals this year, and for Dr.'s Kate Atchley and Cheryl Barksdale for their inspiration and teachings on organizational culture. I wish I could have spent more time with this team.

I am grateful to my Finance Professor, Dr. Philip Daves for having loads of patience with my excel skills and not kicking me off the bus for not knowing there were formulas in Excel! ☺, and Laura Cole, PhD for her patient tutoring of the finance sessions. Thank goodness I sat next to Koji Sparks, MD MBA, on the first day of Finance, and his kindness explaining what Dr. Daves was doing with the excel spreadsheet! I think I aged 10 years that day!

I am grateful to have spent a wonderful year with my 49 classmates in the PEMBA program. The bonds and support I developed with my cohort group of Kevin Trice, MD MBA, Mike Ponder, MD MBA, and Rami Saydjari, MD MBA was memorable. I can't count the number of times they helped answer my "dumb" questions. ☺

"PEMBA-50", "one team, one goal" was our class motto. Thank you all for allowing me to be your classmate.

Richard

INTRODUCTION

Our organization sponsor for the Lean process improvements, Dr. Peter Bath, was a regular presence for most of our Lean brainstorming meetings. I think he describes best what we accomplished in our Lean project when he stated,

"What started with an innocent question about engineering and efficiencies soon turned into a structured approach to lean analysis and efficiencies with team meetings, coaching sessions, and moments of celebration. The operating theaters in which we spend much of our professional life are a worthy setting for this study. Professional interests and eagerness of our bariatric surgeon and his surgical team made the study not only meaningful but also enjoyable. Our team has demonstrated effectively how throughput time into specific dimensions of the surgical flow can be significantly reduced and sustained. This project, as all projects, went through the traditional cycle of forming, storming, norming, and performing. Moments of group discussion unlocked potential solutions, and scope of responsibility were very carefully discussed and enabled to proceed given the underlying trust between all parties."

"To have a Lean project that is successful, engaging, empowering, and inspiring to the members of the surgical department is remarkable. The good work of the anesthesia team in partnership with our bariatric team has inspired other surgeons and their teams to ask, 'When is our turn'?"

Lean Thinking

"The principles of value and value stream are part of Lean thinking defined by Womack and Jones and are an integral component of the Toyota philosophy in auto production. The Toyota way addresses similar issues in healthcare. For both Toyota and the Surgery Clinic, the basic idea is to provide what is needed, at the time it is needed and where it is needed."

Business Case

Our Team set out to measure and reduce the time interval between our surgeon's completion of one operation and his incision in the subsequent procedure; we continually reviewed how our actions reduced this idle time for our surgeon, always keeping in mind our ultimate objective of a 20-minute time improvement for each surgery. If we can accomplish this goal, then in a typical 8 hour work day, composed of 4 X 2 hour procedures, we gain over an additional hour in OR capacity.

Improved effectiveness leads to an opportunity to add over one more hour of operating room capacity per eight hour shift per OR, 2X week = 100-130 hours per year. Contribution margin @ $800/hr. = $80,000-$100,000 per year for our Team; possible reduction in OT expense of $10,000 per year for our Team.

A SURGEON'S PERSPECTIVE

By: John Dietrick, M.D. FACS,

Director, Bariatric Surgery Program,

Florida Hospital Tampa

I am in a unique position as the surgeon in "Room 6" where the process of change is taking place. I have tried on numerous previous occasions to "change the system" in order to realize a more efficient day. However, to make this change appears self-serving and is akin to "moving a mountain". I finally settled in to accept the status quo and work within the boundaries of my environment until Dr. Silver asked for my help with the Lean 6 Sigma project. For me, efficiency means less time spent between operations (from when an operation is complete to when the next operation starts). And while I can keep myself busy making rounds and doing paperwork between procedures, there can be a fair amount of wasted or "down" time between operations. So it goes without saying that I am a ready participant.

I have a few observations regarding the process of change. First, the employees who work directly with me, such as the first assistant, the scrub nurse and the circulator are truly excited about making changes. These are the individuals who are responsible, or blamed, for any excessive amount of time between operations. They know why there is inefficiency in the system and have solutions to this. Yet they know, as I do, that numerous other individuals and even other departments impact their workflow. They are anxious for a change in order to make their work more efficient and for it to "make sense". Yet they also know that this will require the cooperation of many other employees.

A second observation is the amount of pride and dedication that the employees have in their jobs when senior leadership is listening to their opinions. They become engaged and excited about making changes for the sake of "a better product". They will readily share ideas, take on extra tasks and stay late to solve problems.

A final observation is the resistance of some employees to embrace the process of change. It is my opinion that change presents an element of risk. These employees may sense the risk of loosing a job or of a position of leadership. They may also benefit from the status quo. It is ironic that their very reluctance to change increases the risk to their job.

It was recommended that I make a change to one of the patterns of workflow that I had been doing for as long as I have been in practice. It is interesting to me that, while I completely understand and am willing to make that change, I have a tendency to revert to the previous pattern of work that I was used to. I have to remind myself to make a left instead of a right. And while I sometimes rationalize to myself that it really doesn't make a difference, I make that change because I know how important it is to the team and how much of a team process our work truly is. / John Dietrick, MD

OUR STORY

Context

❖ Florida Hospital Tampa, a non-profit community hospital, has recently become part of a large multi-hospital organization run by the Adventist Health System.

❖ The campus is located in the northern Tampa Bay region with over 400 licensed beds.

❖ There are close to 20,000 surgical procedures performed per year in approximately 30 operating and procedure rooms at the Tampa campus.

❖ The Pepin Heart Center, Women's Center, Outpatient Surgery Center, Endoscopy, and Main Operating Room contain most of the surgical procedures performed on campus.

❖ "Team 6" is the surgical team at Florida Hospital Tampa leading the way on a Lean process improvement in the operating rooms.

Challenge

❖ ↓ Cycle time or "circuit time" (time that surgeon is not cutting) leading to ↑ Surgeon productivity

❖ ↑ Employee engagement, empowerment, and productivity

❖ ↓ Wasted time leading to ↑ OR Capacity

❖ ↑ Surgeon satisfaction

Opportunity

* ↓ "Circuit Time" (time surgeon is idle) by decreasing:

  1) In OR to cut time +

  2) Surgery End- to leave OR time interval +

  3) "Wheels-out to wheels-in" (leave OR until return to OR for next case) time interval

* ↓ "Wheels-out to Wheels-in" ='s 40% of "circuit time"

* ↓ In OR to cut time ='s 45% of circuit time

* ↓ Surgery end to leave OR = 15% circuit time

* Opportunity to add 1 more hour of operating room capacity per 8 hour shift per OR, 2x week for our team = ↑ contribution margin to hospital

* Our team has improved cycle time by 16% for all of Dr. Dietrick's surgeries, and 20% for his laparoscopic band procedures.

* ↓ Cycle time produced by our team = potential ↑ OR capacity → $80,000 potential revenue for the team, or

* ↓ Potential overtime expense = $10,000/yr. for the team

* Multiply potential ↑ capacity for 10 teams = potential $800,000 added revenue, or $100,000 potential overtime expense reduction

* Goal: Our team has set a goal for an additional ↓ cycle time for all surgeries of 16%, and 10% for all laparoscopic band procedures = ↑ potential revenue/ savings > $100,000 for our Team!

HOW TO BEGIN

The initial design of the process improvement for a Lean operating room includes defining the project with a charter. An example of our organizational goals and initiatives at Florida Hospital Tampa was created as follows:

Project Name	Dr. Dietrick "Team 6" Lean Initiative
Location	Main Operating Room "6"
Team Leader	Dr. John Dietrick
Sponsor	Dr. Peter Bath
Facilitator	Dr. Richard Silver
Team 6	Dr. Dietrick, Dr. Beckenstein, Chris Weber, RN, Rick Gonzalez, FA, Yudit Conrado, CST, Mary Horsman, CRNA, Jackie VanCleave, AA-C
Lean Consultants	Michael Gilkey, JD Nicholle Henning, RN
Project Description/Mission	Measure, improve, and establish model for improved efficiency for all OR's
Business Case	Opportunity to add over one more hour of operating room capacity per eight hour shift per OR, 2X week=100-130 hours per year. Contribution margin @ $800/hr.=$80,000-$100,000 per year for Team 6; possible reduction in OT expense $10,000 per year for Team 6

Deliverables	"CIRCUIT TIME":
	1. ↓ "Room to Induction" time by 9 minutes from baseline resulting in a 20 minute time interval
	2. ↓ "Wheels out-Wheels in" time by12 minutes leading to a 15 minute time interval ·
	3. ↓ Surgery end- to room out time by 3 minutes leading to an 8 minute time interval
GOALS/METRICS	The desired outcome is a 30% reduction in cycle time from 65-68 minutes to 43- 45 minutes per Team 6 surgical procedure ▯ > 1 hour saved per 8 hour shift
PROCESS AND OWNER	The processes affected by this project are Dr. Dietrick's surgical procedures. The owners of the process are Team 6 members.
PROJECT SCOPE IS	Reduction in wasted time/Surgeon's ability to add more to block time; reduction in overtime expense. Increase in revenue for hospital.
Project Start	June 2011

MILESTONES:	**July 13:** Review Time Study: 1st Organizational Meeting
	July 20: Gemba Walk Lean term defined as a means of gathering real-time, first-hand information on the status of the production process by walking around the plant and observing what is happening).
	July 21: Team 6 Presentation to Entire OR
	July 25: Team 6 Brainstorm: Anesthesia to take patient in room, track calls to Surgical Nursing Assistants (SNA's), track incomplete trays
	July 27: Begin July 25 suggestions. Continue time study/brainstorm sessions
	August-November: weekly or bi-weekly brainstorm sessions, report progress. Ongoing: Create standard work document, review video study of team in OR-repeat study-wide angle lens

"CIRCUIT TIME"

Operating room time is expensive. Our goal is to maximize surgery time leading to an increase contribution margin for our hospital. We approached the goal by trying to decrease the time intervals of the 3 components of the surgeon's idle time("Circuit Time"):

1. ↓ Time interval between entering the operating room ("Wheels-in") and surgical incision ("First cut") = 45% of "circuit time"

2. ↓Time interval between surgery end → patient leaving the operating room = 15% of "circuit time"

3. ↓"Wheels out-wheels in"; the time interval between one patient leaving the operating room → the next patient entering the operating room = 40% of "circuit time"

We believe monitoring and improving the above 3 metrics provides the best opportunity to maximize our surgeons' time as a result of all team members working together.

Focusing solely on turnover time only addresses approximately 40% of the circuit time. Better integration of surgeon, anesthesia, and operating room teams occurs when all 3 time intervals are decreased by teamwork.

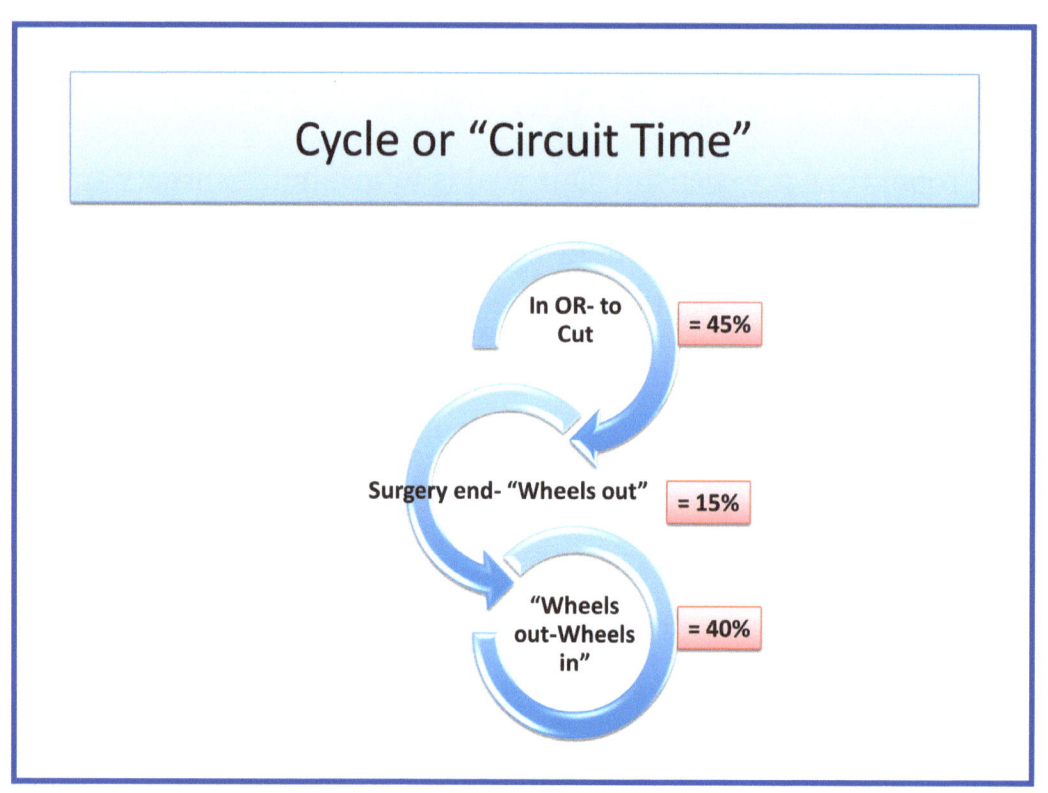

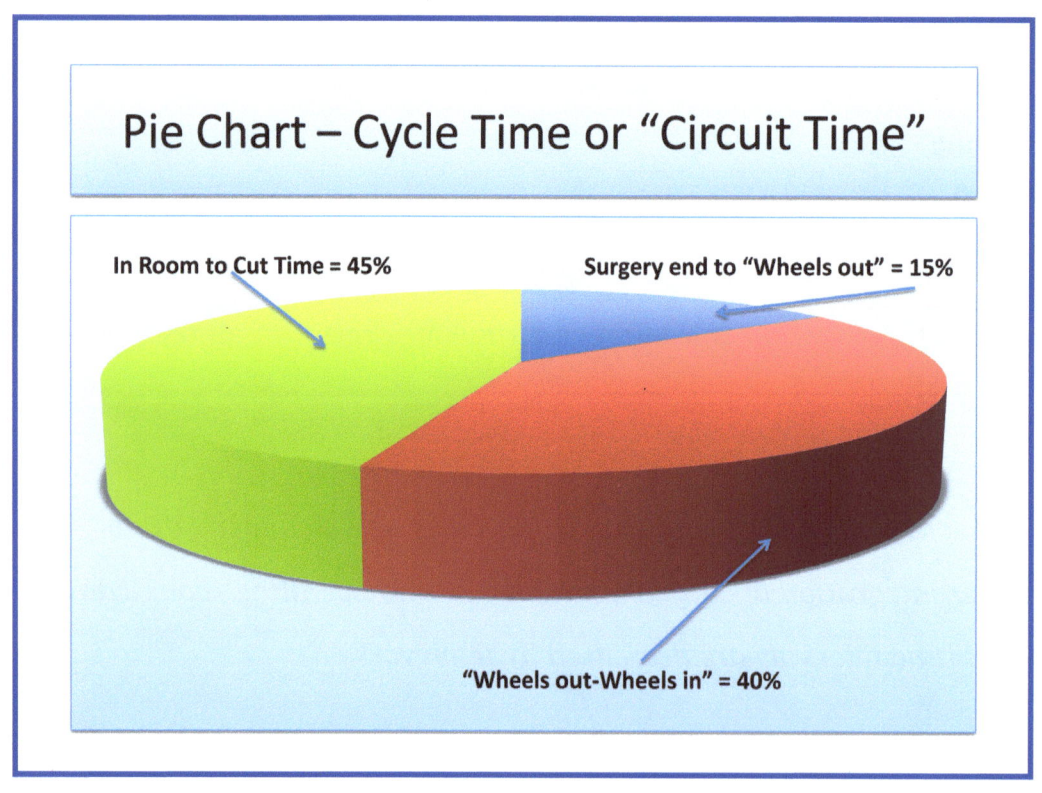

WAYS TO DECREASE "CIRCUIT TIME"

1. Reduction of the time interval between surgery completion and the patient leaving the operating room

Requirements:

* Surgical Nursing Assistant (SNA) availability and wireless communication for rapid response with the OR team
* SNA ready and waiting for OR team
* Anesthesia team understanding details and sequence of surgeon's routine-allows for efficient timing and dosing of anesthetic agents—timely awakening and exiting the operating room

2. Reduction of the time interval between the Patient entering the operating room ("Wheels in") and incision

Requirements:

* Surgeon presence and assistance when patient enters the OR, and ready to operate at completion of patient prep and drape with no delay waiting for the "time out"
* Anesthesia care team focuses on patient during induction and intubation while OR team prepares room for surgery
* All prep and shave supplies in room
* Surgeon washes hands while patient is prepped
* Case cart instruments and supplies for the following procedure organized in close proximity to operating room with complete instrument sets.

3. Reduction of the time interval, "Wheels out-Wheels-in"

Requirements:

- OR team begins organizing cleaning process prior to patient leaving operating room
- Organized, fully stocked cleaning cart for SNA use
- SNA to OR with organized cart, preferably in a team of two.
- "Team 6" assists SNA with room turnover
- Circulator assists scrub tech and first assist, while anesthesia team transports the patient to the OR
- Linens stored in room
- Availability of special equipment (harmonic scalpel, bookwalter)
- Wireless communication device for circulator to contact anesthesia and other needed assistance

"THE TEAM"

A fundamental philosophy for our project is to empower our operating team members to feel valued, respected, and relied on for input. Traditional organizations rely on dictums from above, with little input or explanations from those doing the actual work. We have created a framework to develop an organizational process improvement based on inputs and brainstorming suggestions from our team. We discovered that listening to and supporting suggestions from our team members was key to our success; this is illustrated in the following diagram:

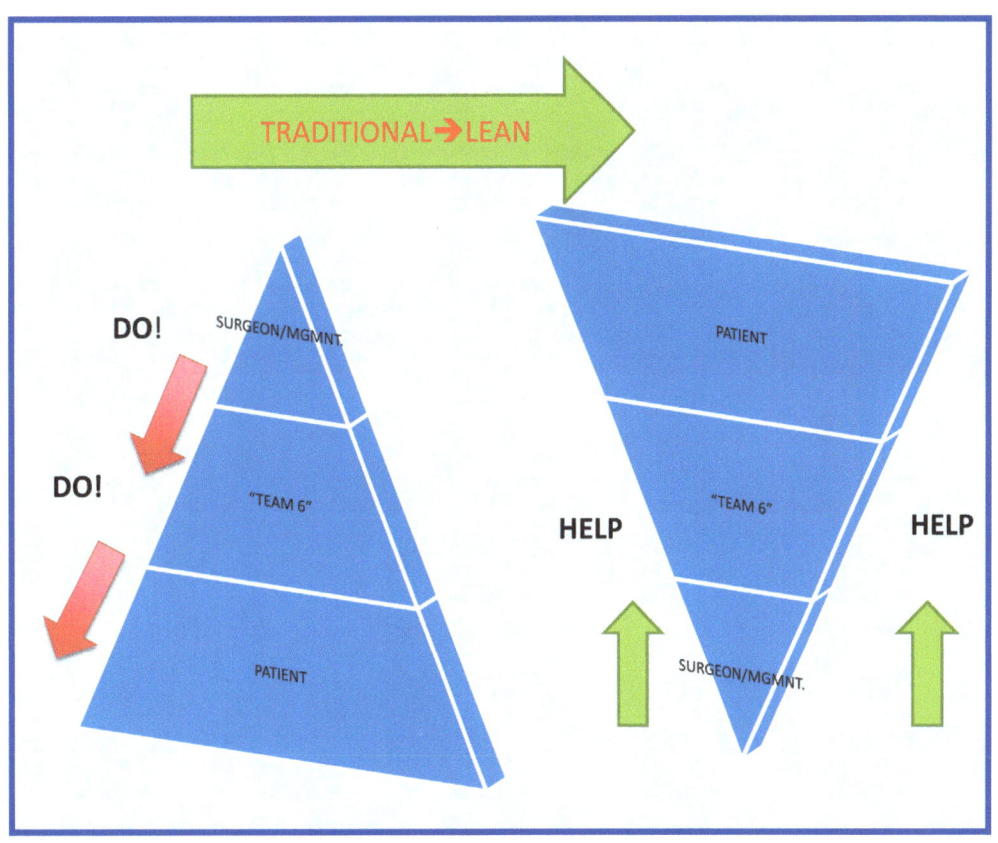

DEDICATED TEAMS

MAXIMIZING EFFECTIVENESS

Fundamental to our Lean flow study was a dedicated team ("Team 6"), consisting of surgeon, anesthesia care team, operating room team, and ancillary support. We believe with this model, wasted time looking for personnel and equipment is minimized. Team members cooperate, understand their process, and maximize efficiency. Each team member recognizes his or her role. Wasted time searching for personnel and equipment is reduced. The "old way" and "new way" of functioning is shown in the following picture with members of the OR team wasting time looking for people and supplies versus everyone team members being in the right place at the right time.

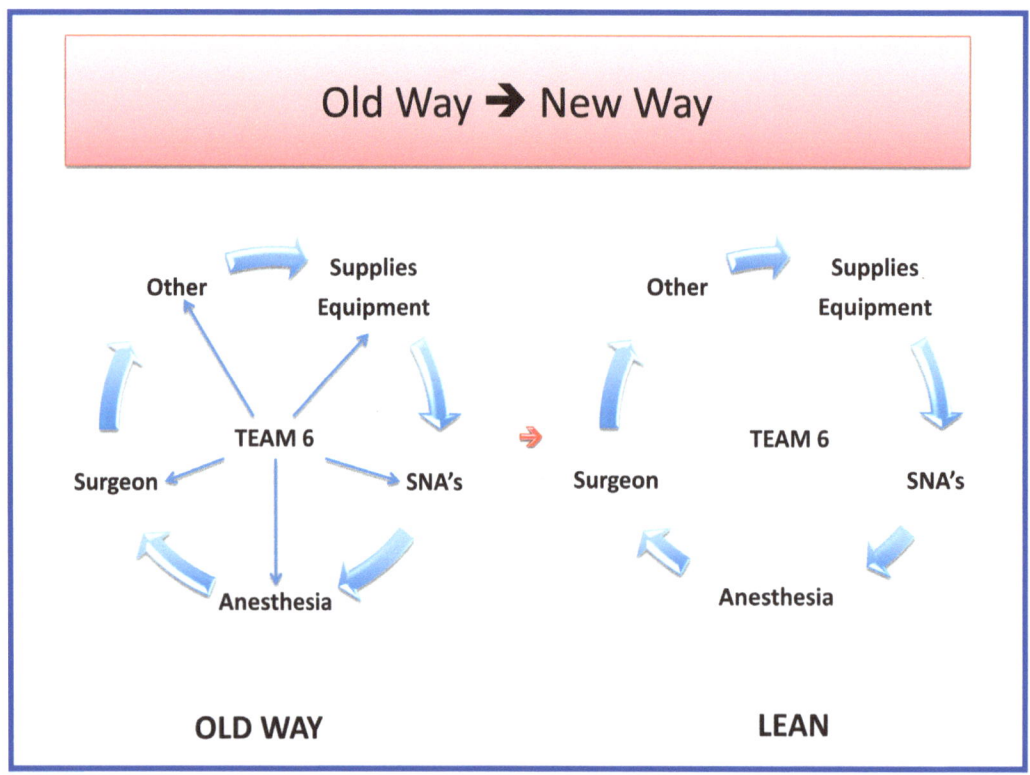

Our plan is for all members of the OR team to function as an efficient unit, minimizing time spent hunting for team members and supplies. Our goal is to have:

1) Shared objectives

2) Shared awareness of the process

3) Constant Lean application to identify opportunities

4) Constant attention to simplify, ↓ waste.

DEDICATED ANESTHESIA TEAM

The dedicated anesthesia team positively impacts patient flow in all 3 segments of the "Circuit Time":

1. Reduction in the time interval from surgery completion until patient leaves the operating room. Familiarity with the surgeon's routine enables the anesthesia care team to efficiently manage the emergence from anesthesia and avoid prolonged anesthesia emergence.

2. "Wheels out-wheels in" is reduced as the anesthesia team transports the patient to the operating room allowing the circulator more time assisting the OR team prepare for the next patient. Good communication is necessary between the circulating nurse and the anesthesia team for success in this routine.

3. When the anesthesia team brings the patient to the OR, the "wheels-in" to incision time is reduced because the circulating nurse is parallel processing with anesthesia.

DEDICATED SURGEON CHAMPION AND TEAM

A committed surgeon and his or her dedicated team are fundamental to the Lean process improvement. Dr. Dietrick and his team followed these basic principles:

❖ The surgeon is present and assists his team with patient positioning.

❖ The surgeon is present and ready to start surgery simultaneously with the completion of the patient prep and drape.

❖ At the completion of an operation, our surgeon finalizes the necessary steps for the next patient as his first priority. This is an important step because the circulator is able to do his or her safety check in an efficient manner following the surgeon's visit and return to the operating room to assist the team for the next case.

ANALYSIS TOOL: "PDSA"

One of the tools we utilized for our team process improvement is a Plan-Do-Study-Act (PDSA) sequence, also known as the Deming Cycle.

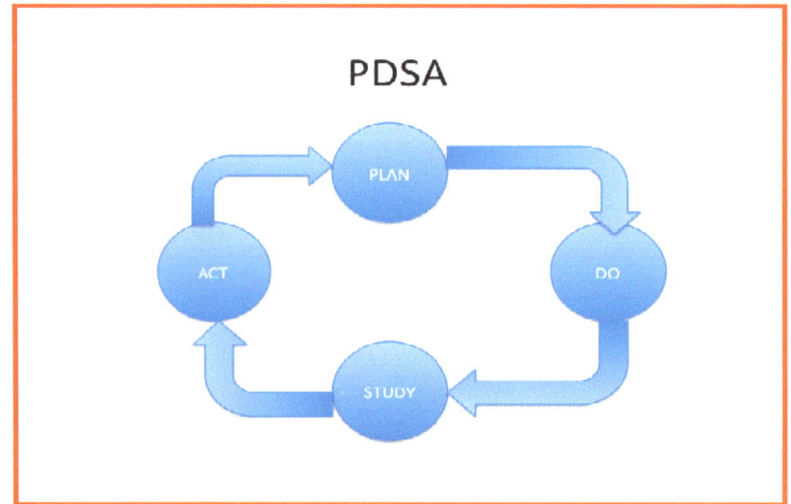

PLAN

During the Plan stage we brainstormed how to improve our surgeon's efficiency. We determined the process to be improved was the "circuit time". An improvement goal was set at 15- 20 minutes per surgery. The changes to be implemented were scheduled to begin as soon as possible. We planned to measure the effects of our changes daily, and report the results monthly. As previously described, our initial plan included surgeon and anesthesia parallel processing with the operating room team.

DO

In the DO stage we informed our surgeon the process improvement was ready to begin. Our team (team 6) was identified, and buy-in was established. Next, we made our changes, and our circulating nurse began the measurements needed for the study phase. Through weekly brainstorming sessions we monitored our changes, and continually tried to improve our time intervals.

STUDY

During the Study stage we reviewed data collected in the previous DO stage. We reviewed how much our process improved, always keeping in mind an ultimate objective of approximately 15 to 20 minute time improvement.

ACT

During the ACT stage, we began the changes agreed upon in the DO stage. We considered new proposals as we cycled back to the PLAN stage. Planning occurred during the regular brainstorming sessions, usually on a weekly or bi-weakly interval. We continually looked for ways to tweak different areas for improvement as the cycle returned to the planning stage. As much as possible, we requested feedback from our surgeon/customer for new opportunities. Improvements were standardized as much as possible. One of our mantras was to improve our efficiency without requesting additional financial support. Furthermore, at no time was there ever talk of reducing staff as our efficiency improved!

SUSTAIN

To sustain the process we held regular meetings with continued monitoring of the Lean process improvement. More importantly, the team members' perspectives were always sought for suggestions and recommendations. The team members are an important driving force for ongoing improvement.

MEASURE PROGRESS

We discovered regular review of our time studies to be an invaluable part of the project. A log of the time intervals of the "circuit time" was kept daily and presented during each brainstorm session. The graphs and charts provided a visual summary of the team's progress. Examples of our charts for all "Team 6" surgeries, as well as only laparoscopic bands, are pictured below:

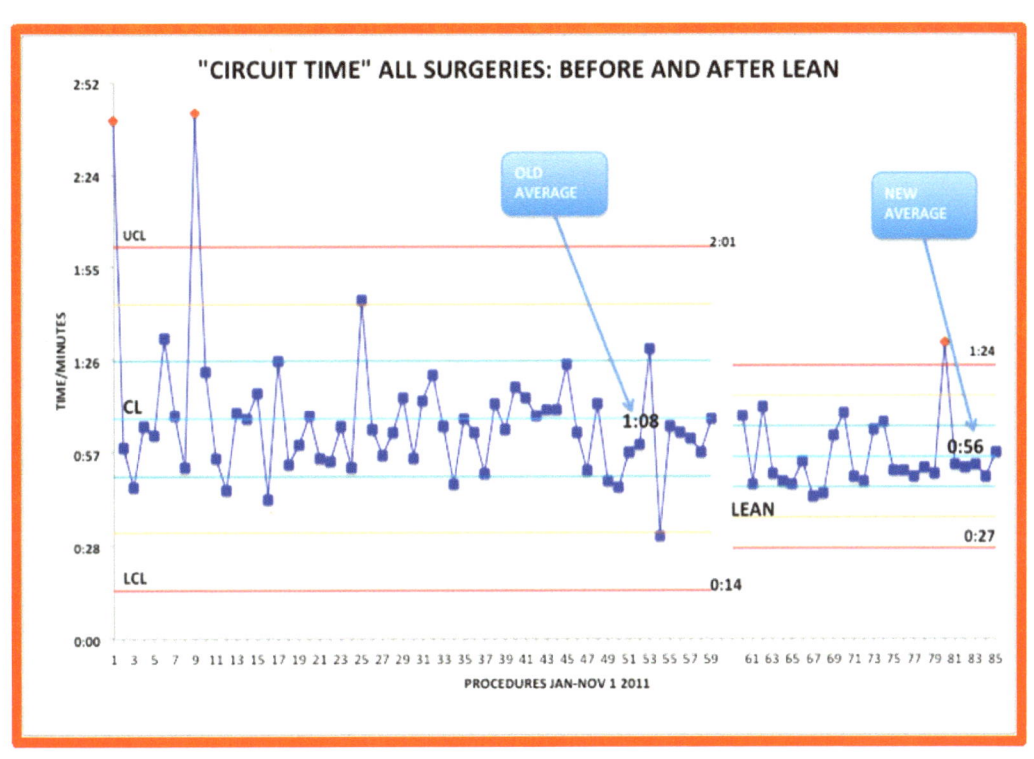

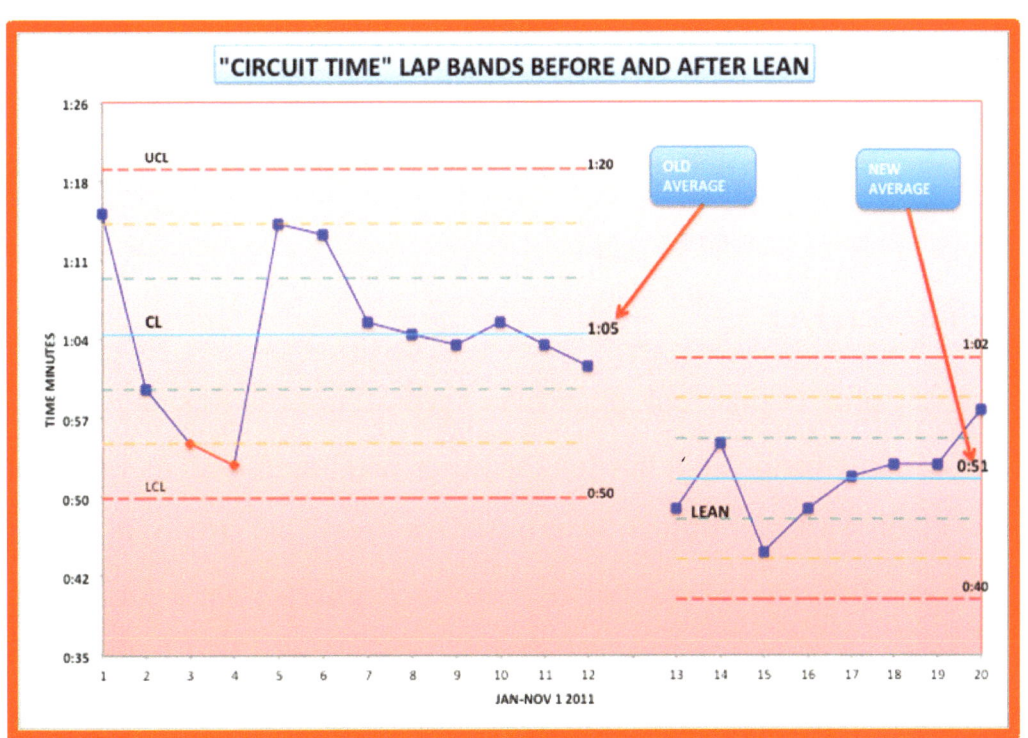

29.

TEAM ENGAGEMENT: TESTIMONIALS

"TEAM 6" SCRUB TECH

By Yudit Conrado, CST

The lean project has meant a lot to me. I have learned a lot about work in a group. We have worked hard and changed the techniques of doing our job many times over. All our efforts have been done for our patients and their safety. We like to think that we have made a difference and that our work is going to help other surgical teams. I would like to thank all the departments that have been working with us to improve our services. The lean project is a process that would never succeed without all the hard working people that have participated. In my opinion, with projects as the lean process, we can improve the costumer services in our facility and be more accurate and organized, which gives us the opportunity of helping more patients. / YC

Yudit Conrado

"TEAM 6" FIRST ASSISTANT

By Rick Gonzalez, FA

The lean study project that took place over several months was an experience to be had, not only for myself, but for the other team members as well. I never knew how much work went into a lean initiative until I got involved. The learning of all of the processes that are involved in preparing a patient for surgery was much more than I expected. I felt it my duty was solely to help prepare the operating room suite of equipment and supplies and assisting in the surgery. But I was wrong.

During the study, I learned how many pieces of the preparation puzzle there truly were; from registration to preoperative testing, preoperative holding to the operating room, and then anesthesia to recovery. This process has involved many aspects of medical care and I soon realized how a slow down in just one area can eventually change the outlook for the entire day. Flow is key!

But consistent flow is what we were trying to achieve. Practice makes perfect, but I soon came to realize how imperfect the process was. Though working with the team for over 4 years has brought a comfort level there was much room for improvement. Just one change in our regular routine has improved the process dramatically. Keeping that change and looking into the next can bring greater efficiency into our processes while maintaining a safe environment for our patients.

I look forward to participating in this process as we distribute our research throughout the operating room and involve other participants. I would like to thank our team 6 members: Dr. John Dietrich, Chris Webber RN, Yudit Conrado CST, as well as Peter Bath, Mission Vice President, Florida Hospital Tampa, and Dr. Richard Silver, Director, Lean Methods to Improve Operating Room Throughput-a Multidisciplinary Team Approach. / RG
Rick Gonzalez, FA

"TEAM 6" CIRCULATING NURSE

By Chris Weber, RN

When I was asked to participate in the lean study, I was eager to do so. I just knew that our team, a strong, well bonded team, would prove that our process would not need to change much, because "This is the way we have always done it. How can it get much better?" What I did not see coming was the opportunity to look into all the processes of the other departments we work with. This enabled us to re-assess the way we have always done it and clear up some of the frustrations that have bogged up our efficiency.

On the heels of a highly publicized mission completed by the United States Navy SEAL Team 6, we gave ourselves a name, Team 6, named after our OR room number. After joining the US Navy upon graduating high school, I learned quickly to appreciate cohesiveness as a team first hand, working with helicopter pilots and aircrew, training for various missions. Being familiar with the Navy team concept from working in a helicopter squadron, this principle has never been forgotten and will always ring true to me. This team name gave us a sense of pride and an identity.

Through the rigors of data collection, meetings, and changes in routines, the deeper assessment proved to me that there was still room to grow, and change is inevitable always.

I think this study has brought visibility not only to us, one OR team, but to our whole department. We have been blessed by having support from administration on this endeavor. Through this project, we have brought attention globally to deficiencies in our unit. Streamlining our processes and bringing attention to resources we need in order to be successful has been accomplished. I thoroughly enjoy having a hand in such a worthy project, and look forward to the days ahead for more growth. / CW

Chris Weber, RN circulator

Team 6

SURGICAL NURSING ASSISTANTS (SNA'S)

"Since they have started the team 6 project, I have noticed several changes that have improved efficiency for the operating room. Quite a few suggested ideas have been implemented so far. This whole project has put me in a more positive frame of mind. I look forward to more and better changes in the future."/ Roger

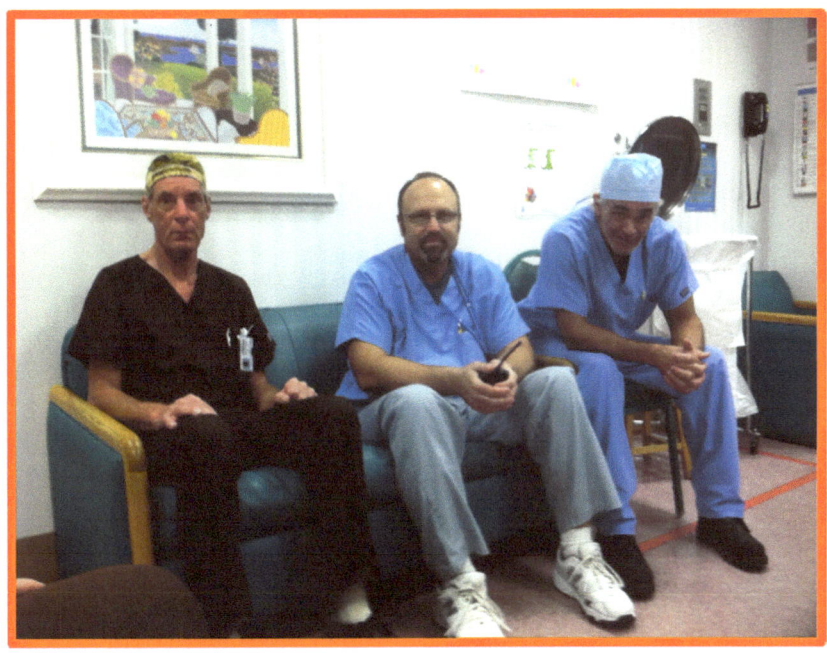

Left to Right: Roger Vandergilder, Brian Hensley, Dennis Moore: "Early Bird" SNA's

OPERATING ROOM MANAGER

Thank you for your hard work on this.

Rhonda Hawks, RN

The team 6 turnover project has created a sense of camaraderie among the operating room staff and the anesthesia department. This had been a true team effort and we have seen a significant decrease in our turnover times. The other team members within the department are anxious to begin their own team and this has created a type of "friendly competition" among the staff with each OR team wanting to have the best turnover times.

Having everyone involved, including SNAs as well as the circulator, scrub, surgeon and first assistant has heightened the team effort.

Management is excited to move forward with utilizing this standard to decrease overall turnovers and increase physician satisfaction. / RH

DIRECTOR OF SURGICAL SERVICES

Our Journey to Perioperative Excellence

Martha Kent RN MS CNOR

Providing excellence in Perioperative environment centers on a focus of our key customers: patients, surgeons and anesthesia providers and surgical team members. Daily initiatives that enhance the patient experience and outcomes include the Surgical Care Improvement Project (SCIP) core measures, compliance with National Patient Safety Goals (NPSG) and ensuring surgeon and team member satisfaction and engagement. A central thread to satisfaction for all key customers and the goal of perioperative excellence is patient throughput and efficiencies. Continually improving our product and connecting our teams to purpose is key to market growth.

In June and July of 2009 key team members in Surgical Services and Registration participated in workout sessions to identify opportunities to improve patient throughput. With the teams suggestions action plans were defined and processes were begun to enhance and measure throughput with the focus on first case start times and turnover times. Improvement goals were attained with first case start times increasing from sixty nine percent to eighty six percent and turnover time decreasing from an overall average of thirty-two minutes down to twenty- eight minutes. As the surgical teams worked on continually improving turnover time and physicians engaged in first case start time improvements positive physician feedback was received as the team efforts and enthusiasm had begun to create results.

As our teams continued to focus on these two goals an invitation was presented for a team to participate in a lean workout project and Team 6 was formed. Team members included the anesthesia providers, the Surgeon, Registered Nurse (RN) Circulator, Certified Surgical First Assistant (CFA) and Certified Surgical Technician (CST) from the advanced laparoscopic specialty. The number of team members was intentionally kept small, as a small test of change was the goal. Team brainstorming and mapping of current state processes was key to identifying waste as was partnering with the Sterile Processing Department.

Additionally I would like to share some observations from our weekly communication meetings as Team 6 became Lean Team 6 and the project progressed. What made this small test of change different from our prior action plans is what I would like to describe as the 5E's: empowerment, engagement, energy, excitement, and exceptional commitment to success and excellence. The team successes and data were communicated to physicians at medical staff meetings and to our surgical teams at staff meetings. Requests to participate and implement the identified lean process changes were coming from other specialty teams and surgeons asking "when will they be able to implement the process changes, when is it our turn?" The phenomenon of friendly competition had developed as teams became engaged and commitment to improving efficiency became contagious. Fundamental to success of the throughput efficiency initiatives is participation and engagement of the anesthesia providers.

Implementation planning and sustainability of the identified turnover efficiency gains describes the current state of this project. Our journey to Perioperative Excellence and patient throughput is not simply a stated goal; it is defined by a culture and attitude of engagement by all. /MK

MY PERSONAL REFLECTION

I was fortunate to develop an excellent and professional connection with our bariatric surgeon, Dr. John Dietrick, and his operating room team. The affiliation has lead to an opportunity to develop a Lean model for all operating rooms. An empowered team and surgeon buy-in led to an exciting study with significant results. Most importantly, we are developing a Lean model that will eventually be shared with other operating room teams.

Along the way, not all was smooth sailing. I made mistakes and was occasionally bruised. I want to share the lessons I learned in the following 10 Commandments for Lean:

DR. SILVER'S TEN COMMANDMENTS FOR A LEAN PROCESS IMPROVEMENT

1. ENGAGE AN IMPORTANT AND HIGH-RANKING MEMBER OF YOUR HOSPITAL ADMINISTRATION IN THE LEAN PROCESS.

There are multiple groups to deal with when championing a Lean operating room process. Top-level hospital administrators prioritize safety and customer care. Dr. Peter Bath played the important role of "leveling the playing field" and being the "glue" with our process improvement.

2. EMPOWER ALL MEMBERS OF THE TEAM TO PROVIDE INPUT AND POSSESS EQUAL VOICE.

An important aspect of our process improvement involved allowing equal voice and equal participation by all team members. Those workers involved in the daily functioning of our operating rooms are frequently those with the best ideas for improving efficiency. To maintain the team's focus and sustainability requires constant listening to and validating all team members. In our case, the circulating nurse, first assist, and scrub tech were important contributors to our regular meetings.

3. DO NOT BLAME OR "POINT FINGERS".

Starting a process improvement requires teambuilding not team destruction. When starting a process improvement for an operating room, people become defensive. We established, at the beginning, a ground rule of no blame or finger pointing. We firmly believe better results are achieved with open minds and a "no blame" attitude.

4. DON'T TAKE SETBACKS PERSONALLY.

When trying to introduce a Lean initiative, there will be those for, against, and neutral. Don't be discouraged if 100% support is not obvious from day one.

5. RESPECT EQUALLY ALL TEAM MEMBERS.

Introducing a lean operating room process improvement involves team members of various ranks. To ensure continued success, each team member must feel equally important regardless of status or position within the organization. We treat all team members the same, regardless of status, and it has been critical in maintaining enthusiasm, support, and involvement.

6. FOCUS ON QUALITY AND EFFICIENCY.

During our project we never rushed to save time. Our overarching philosophy was to improve efficiency without compromising safety. Our team members would often marvel at how the operating room times were improving without any need to rush or compromise safety and quality.

7. SURGEON SUPPORT AND ENCOURAGEMENT IS KEY.

The importance of an involved surgeon is paramount. We were fortunate during our 1st process improvement to have Dr. Dietrick, a very supportive surgeon, actively involved in improving our system.

8. SIMPLIFY AS MANY STEPS AS POSSIBLE.

There are many components to a smooth running operating room team. Our goal was to always simplify and reduce unnecessary steps.

9. VALUE ALL TEAM MEMBERS' TIME.

Brainstorming sessions were held after routine work hours. Team members often had other commitments and could not attend. We respected those obligations.

10. IT'S ALL ABOUT THE PATIENT.

It's important to remember the patient is the ultimate beneficiary of all we are trying to improve.

CONCLUSIONS

Surgeon/Anesthesia/ OR Team Contribution

I believe the role performed by anesthesia, the surgeon and his team in our Lean initiative made a positive impact in improving efficiency. In the spaghetti diagram below, our circulator is traced during a turnover time period between laparoscopic band and laparoscopic cholecystectomy procedures. The turnover time was 16 minutes without rushing. There was minimal wasted motion for the circulator as the surgeon saw his next surgical patient as first priority, and the anesthesia team brought the patient to the OR.

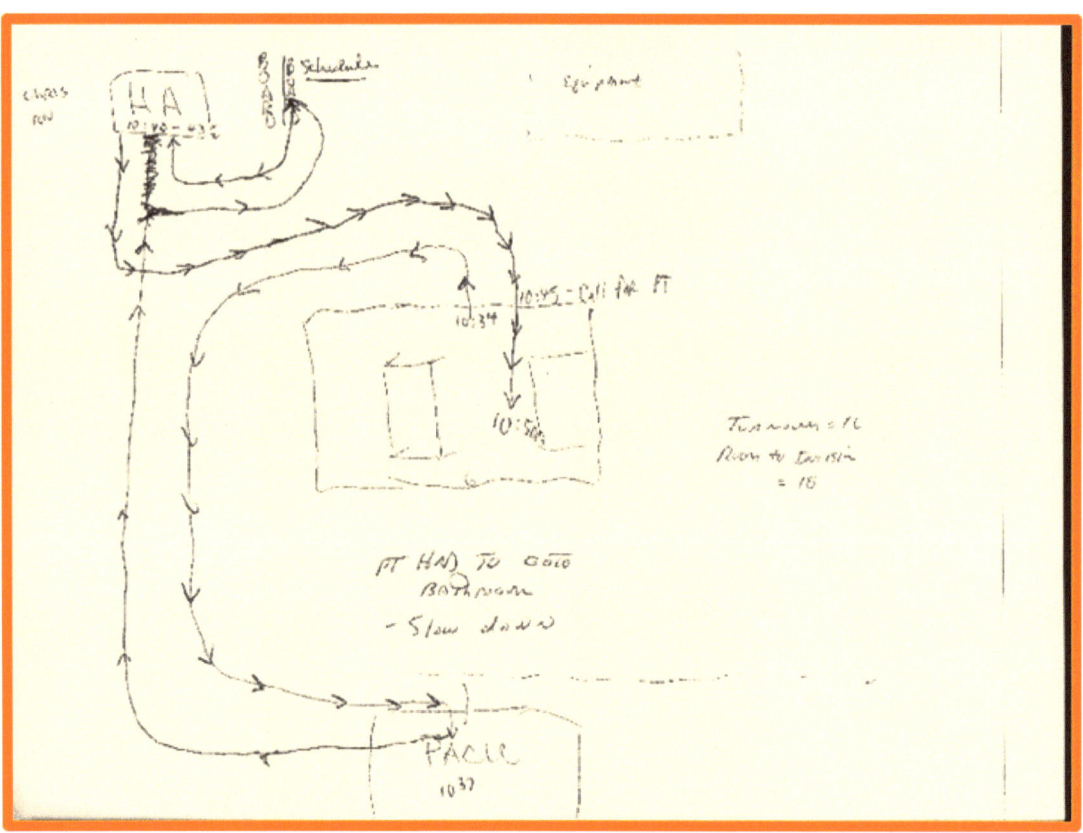

Exciting Opportunities

The Lean initiative for the Bariatric Program is an exciting opportunity to introduce and develop a Lean process for other operating room teams. I believe focusing on one team with short-term wins, or rapid process improvements (RPI's), enables us to share our Lean experience with other teams. At the time of this writing, there is interest to expand a Lean initiative to other teams.

15-20% Improvement

The bariatric process has evolved into a significant and important project for our healthcare organization. Our team is developing a lean model upon which the entire surgery program may benefit. We have been studying and implementing process improvements for almost 6 months. We have been fortunate to have many individuals working together. We have an engaged hospital sponsor and enthusiastic surgeon, anesthesia and OR team. We have demonstrated an average 15 to 20% time reduction for team 6's "circuit time." We continue to meet regularly, brainstorm, test, and implement suggestions. We have determined our future state goals. We take our project seriously as we want the process to be sustainable in the long run and successful for the entire operating room.

Goals

One of our goals will be to continue to seek ways to improve the non-operative throughput for our surgeons and patients. Another one of our goals is to do more with less. So far, our performance improvements have succeeded with no increase in costs per case.

Future

Cendan demonstrated in a study of operating room efficiency, interdisciplinary workflow redesign might result in additional cases being completed each day. Although we are not at this juncture in our study, we ultimately hope to increase operating room procedures secondary to improved efficiency. In an increasingly resource-constrained environment, efficiency is critical for maintaining access to quality care. Surgeons, nurses, and operating room (OR) administrators often turn to new technologies to help solve this problem. Improving efficiency in the OR, however, is often dependent on synchronizing functions of key personnel from nursing, anesthesia, and surgery rather than on devices that cut, sew, or staple faster.

FINAL SUMMARY

Lean techniques are powerful tools to improve a process. We have attempted to use such tools in our organization.

People

In my opinion, the take-home lesson for a Lean process improvement is not the tools, but the people that use the tools. The enthusiasm demonstrated by the members of team 6 was the main reason for the process improvement in bariatric surgery. The Lean techniques provide a foundation and common vocabulary team members can use to relate to one another.

Sustain

To truly contribute in a major way to our healthcare organization, we will continue to improve on team 6 results and transmit the enthusiasm to other teams. A sustained and significant improvement will require other operating room teams to believe they can make a difference. The real challenge will be in creating a model that will be self sustaining with continued enthusiasm and success.

To sustain will require hard work and continued teambuilding. It will not be enough to paste graphs on hallway walls. Ultimately, we're all working together to create and build an efficient healthcare system we can be proud of.

[i] Womack, JonesDT.LeanThinking.NewYork: Simon and Schuster; 1996.

[ii] Waldhausen et al. Application of Lean methods improves surgical clinic experience. Journal of Pediatric Surgery (2010) 45, 1420-1425.

[iii] Cendan et al, (REPRINTED) ARCH SURG/VOL 141, JAN 2006

[iv] Stahl et al, Surgery June 2006; 717-728

www.ingramcontent.com/pod-product-compliance
Lightning Source LLC
Chambersburg PA
CBHW051103180526
45172CB00002B/758